Pharmaceutical/Medical Representatives
A Mission for Success

A Handbook for Representatives and Managers

By

Travis Doss

ISBN: 1-4033-2825-0 (e-book)
ISBN: 1-4033-2826-9 (Paperback)
ISBN: 1-4033-2827-7 (RocketBook)

Library of Congress Control Number: 2002091830

This book is printed on acid free paper.

Printed in the United States of America
Bloomington, IN

1stBooks - rev. 06/19/02

Foreword

Our generation has been the beneficiary of an explosion of intellectual and medical advances in the treatment of debilitating diseases. It is easy to dwell on the breakthroughs of laboratory scientists and the inspiring efforts of clinical researchers of our era. It is salutary, however, to realize that the greatest pharmacologic breakthrough of all time, the discovery of penicillin by Alexander Fleming, almost came to nothing. Fleming's work was promptly published and widely researched, but despite every medical student's awareness of this miracle drug's wondrous possibilities, millions continued to die on peaceful farms and the trenches of war, of sepsis.

Great efforts were made to enlighten the world of the tremendous promise of this new antibiotic, but since its efficacy was so well known and thereby un-patentable, no company took up the cause of scaling up the drug's production and financing it's distribution.

Indeed, the first patient to demonstrate a dramatic response to penicillin, a British policeman, ultimately died because the lab supplying his doctors with the drug ran out! It took the scourge of a World war to force a consortium of drug companies to work together in Oxford, England, to scale up production and create a distribution plan.

Once this had been achieved, it was assumed the drug that saved so many on the battlefield would be widely adopted throughout the British Isles and beyond. But nothing happened; practitioners, set in their ways, failed to prescribe the life-saving drug despite it's widespread availability. Why, you might ask?

The journals were full of detailed studies demonstrating over and over again the drug's remarkable efficacy. Maybe busy physicians don't read every published article (!). The commercial forces reacted. Glossy advertising, aimed at human doctors, not academic icons, had an immediate impact. The combination of clinical education and shrewd marketing that followed revolutionized the drug industry and the practice of medicine itself. Without any doubt, the evolution of marketing and distribution, combined with professional education, was as much a turning point in our modern medical history as Fleming's first glance at the penicillium mould on his petri dish.

Travis Doss, in this valuable handbook, sets out practical and ethical foundations for success and fulfillment in

Pharmaceutical Marketing and Professional medical education. Doctors respect frankness, honesty, and an effective and reliable product. There is much that a good Pharmaceutical Representative does to ensure ongoing benefit to patients, and our continuing medical advances.

I commend this book as both a practical guide and a spiritual lift, and look forward to working in the years ahead with those who have committed it's principles to practice.

W. E. Sponsel, M.D.

Director, Clinical Research

University of Texas Health Science Center-San Antonio

Acknowledgements

A sincere word of appreciation goes out to all those who generously contributed to the writing of this book by their encouragement, guidance, and voices of approval. Among my many Merck friends and associates, Jim Jones, a partner in Pantheon Partners, Inc., and Jim Jones, Jr., a Business Manager with Merck Human Health, were most helpful in taking the time to critically evaluate the contents of the book, and to share their thoughts from a manager's perspective.

My mentor of recent years, William Eric Sponsel, M.D., has been a real inspiration in his support and suggestions, as I sought a suitable publisher for the book. A special thanks to him for his contribution to the book in the Foreword.

A Mateen Ahmed, Ph.D., President and CEO of New World Medical, Inc., also has been most supportive in his evaluation and analysis of the book. We have discussed the content at length on several occasions, and he has never failed to offer praise, encouragement, and support.

My family, including my wife, Willie, our son and daughter-in-law, Darryl and Anita Doss, and our daughter and son-in-law, Karen and Roger Lee, has been a constant source of support and encouragement. They tell me that they have even used some of the guidelines in my book to obtain better ratings on their performance reviews!

I treasure the contribution my friends, Chuck and Annie Aschenbrenner, made with their careful evaluation and suggestions. Chuck is a former Public School Director of Special Education for the State of Illinois, and Annie is a veteran of hotel management.

The list of contributors would not be complete without acknowledging the unfailing support of my next-door neighbor, Mitchell Davis. Mitchell has a unique perspective on the subject, since he previously operated a medical supply company in Dallas. Having to rely heavily on my years of experience with Merck, I have been concerned that my book might be perceived as a "Merck" book. That is not what I intended, and Mitchell assures me that this is not the case. He believes that any pharmaceutical company could use this book very effectively in their training programs.

My thanks, also, to Don & Cindy Wells for their insight and suggestions from the realm of pharmacy, having owned and operated their own pharmacy for a number of years.

Preface

Relationships have always been an essential element in the performance of a pharmaceutical/medical representative's job. This book is designed to explore those relationships with a variety of people that he/she will find it necessary to relate to. Among these are, 1) the physician, 2) the patient, 3) co-workers, 4) competitors, 5) pharmacists, 6) nurses & assistants, and 7) managers, and perhaps others. From personal experience, the author will describe in considerable detail how each of these groups contribute to the representative's success or failure. He will describe a philosophy that will ultimately lead to sales versus sales as the primary objective.

Personal success will be measured more by how well one handles these relationships. Personal success will lead to sales success, which inevitably will be the primary measure of performance used by management. Considerable discussion also will be devoted to helpful hints that will help new and experienced representatives, as well as managers, derive the greatest benefit from their endeavors.

Table of Contents

Chapter I

Developing a Philosophy From Day One

Patient is Primary Focus

The representative must never lose sight of the fact that the primary focus must always be on the patient, and how he/she can help the healthcare professional provide the best care possible for that patient.

As representatives, we cannot provide treatment to a patient directly. We must seek an understanding of the needs of a patient and relate the utility of our product to those needs. This sounds simple enough, but it's not always that easy. Sometimes a healthcare professional can construct formidable barriers to the achievement of this goal.

Developing a Mutual Respect and Trust

Development of a mutual respect and trust between you and the healthcare professional is a must. This does not always come easy, and may take some time. A review of my first day on the territory best describes what I mean.

Focus Presentation on Patient

After more than a month of intense formal training, I thought I was adequately prepared to carry out my mission for the patient. About mid-afternoon that first day, my District Manager and I set out to make my first call. We picked a clinic that housed ten or twelve doctors of varying specialty. Seeking the office with the least number of patients waiting, we walked into the office of an older OB/GYN doctor. We were politely ushered right in to see the doctor. The doctor was not overly friendly, or even polite, but nevertheless I began my presentation. After a brief period, he pushed his chair back, and in a loud voice said, "What is going on here?" Needless to say, this was rather disturbing to me on my first call. Fortunately, my District Manager, one of the brightest and best the industry has ever produced, came to my rescue. He calmly and politely said, "Doctor, you have the great privilege of being the first doctor that Mr. Doss has ever detailed. Well, he seemed to lighten up a bit after that, and things went much better. He didn't learn much from my first presentation, but I had learned a great deal. In the first place, I was trying to sell my product, rather than focusing on the patient's needs. After a brief introduction, I should have solicited the doctor's participation in establishing his patient's needs. I had not yet established that all important mutual respect and trust.

I found out later that this was, without a doubt, the meanest doctor in town for representatives to call on. He entertained himself by humiliating new and inexperienced representatives. To make my life more miserable, he called all his buddies at the local pharmacies to tell them what a fool he had made of me. I knew my work was cut out for me, so I made a special effort to call on this doctor at regular intervals. I never quite learned to like him, but I do believe we developed that all important mutual trust and respect.

No One Can Make You Feel Inferior Without Your

Permission

I forgot, momentarily, that no one on earth can make you feel inferior without your permission. After that first call, I was ready to seek a new career, but my astute Manager gave me the encouragement I needed to try and see the doctor around the corner of this same clinic.

While we were waiting for our second call, this doctor, a general surgeon/family practitioner, came through the waiting room several times. He had a stern look on his face, looked ten feet tall, and had hands as big as a baseball glove. I was scared to death that I had jumped out of the frying pan into the fire. Before long, he called us back to his office, and low and behold, he was the kindest, most gentle, and gentlemanly person I have ever known.

5

Learning fast from my first call, our discussion this time focused on the needs of the patient, and I was certain I would be rewarded with sales, resulting from this call. The real reward, however, was knowing that I had contributed in some small way to the relief of his patient's pain and suffering.

Our next call in the office next door was on a general surgeon. He wanted to discuss the use of a vitamin K product we had, so he and my District Manager got into a detailed discussion, offering me the opportunity to relax and observe for a few moments.

The doctor was really impressed with my District Manager's grasp of the subject. I found out later that he even impressed his fellow managers. They marveled at the fact that he could even pronounce the word hyperbilirubinemia, without batting an eye!

I have striven all the years of my career to emulate that District Manager, but I don't think I have, until yet, reached his level of expertise and professionalism. You see, he was a true advocate for the representatives he supervised. He listened carefully to what we had to say, and always offered us choices for helping to solve our problems.

About a year later, this particular District Manager was transferred to another District, with greater responsibility. I feel privileged to have shared his wisdom and expertise during that first year. Actually, throughout my career as a pharmaceutical representative, he continued to share his words of wisdom, when we occasionally met at group meetings. Indeed, he shared his helpful thoughts with all representatives, whether under his supervision or not. Unlike many managers, he was not afraid to share his "secrets", if it would benefit the Company as a whole. In other words, he had a good grasp of "the big picture".

I will have more to say later about the profound effect that other managers, as well as associates, have had on my life and career. More also will be said about other managers, and how their techniques helped or hindered my success.

Success and Happiness Are Not Necessarily The Same

Keep in mind that success and happiness are not necessarily the same. It has been said that success is to get what you want. Happiness is to want what you have. It is for that reason that one should always remember the age-old adage that you should be careful what you ask for, you might get it.

Chapter II

The Physician—Developing That All

Important Mutual Trust and Respect

The Focus Is Always On The Patient

Keep in mind that the focus is always on the patient. The physician makes it possible for us to play a role in helping the patient by the physician's use of our products.

The physician bears the sole responsibility for the care of his/her patients, so it is the representative's responsibility to gain an understanding of what the physician feels are his/her patient's needs. Then, and only then, can we present our products in such a way that they offer maximum utility in helping to achieve the physician's objectives.

Interviewing Technique Must Be Skillfully Tactful

It should be emphasized that gaining information about a physician's patients cannot be achieved in an interrogative fashion. To emphasize what I mean, I would suggest you observe the interviewing techniques used by several network news anchors, and ask yourself which technique would be best suited to help you obtain the information you need to tailor your presentation to the needs of the physician and the patient.

I have spent a great deal of time during the course of my career helping train groups of new representatives. During the course of these training sessions, I have frequently played "doctor", for purposes of allowing new representatives to experience fairly realistic practice presentations. One develops a great deal of sympathy for the physician during those early roll play sessions. There are two primary mistakes that occur most frequently in these sessions. One is being too dramatic, or even inaccurate, in the inexperienced representative's description of symptoms. The other is an interrogation that begins immediately, when a representative begins the interview or presentation.

It would behoove all training departments to make sure that each and every trainee has the opportunity to play "doctor" while they are pursuing their basic training. This is the most effective way for a new representative to evaluate his/her own presentation, from the perspective of the physician.

Doctors Sometimes Just Need Someone To Talk To

With a little experience, representatives will realize just how important the development of mutual trust and respect with the physician is. Because of the stress of a large practice, physicians, like most everyone else, will sometimes develop stress-related emotional disorders, such as depression or severe anxiety. Seek help—see a neurologist or psychiatrist, you say. For most people, that is a logical and easy solution. Many physicians do not see it that way. They fear the loss of their practice, and indeed their livelihood, if their patients find out they are seeing a psychiatrist. This is largely unfounded in this day and time, but the fear still exists, just the same. The point is, a physician sometimes just needs someone to talk to— someone that they respect and trust. Frequently, that person is a representative that they have come to feel comfortable with. If this happens to you, be a good listener, and forget about discussing products on that call.

Physicians, like many of their patients, develop very serious diseases, deadly diseases, and it breaks your heart to see them suffer. A couple of instances come to mind. One country doctor, in a small town that I once called on, had dedicated his life to relieving the pain and suffering of his patients. Many are the times, when I would call on this physician in the early morning, he would tell of the patient he had spent the night with at the patient's home. Oftentimes the patient was dying, and he wanted to be there to help, if the patient needed him. One sad day, I called on him again in the early morn, and this time he was the one in need of help. He had just been diagnosed with pancreatic cancer. The next time I saw him was a few weeks later at his funeral.

This was a doctor, who could seat a patient beside his desk, look into their eyes, and tell more about that patient than all the lab tests in the World would show. He had a treatment table, but seldom used it. He was very serious about his practice, and made the most of modern-day medicine. Everyone who knew him, loved him, and he was sorely missed by that community.

The other instance that comes to mind was an internist in my headquarters town. This physician was not a fellowship trained cardiologist, but knew more about cardiology than most of those who claimed to be cardiologists. I learned a lot from this physician on keeping the primary focus on the patient. If my products could truly satisfy a need of his patients, he rewarded me with extensive use of those products.

One day, I walked into this doctor's office, and his nurse told me that he would see me for a minute, but he had a doctor's appointment for himself in a little while. I sensed immediately that something was seriously wrong, so we had a brief personal visit. I wished him well, and he left immediately. His nurse told me confidentially that he, also, had been diagnosed with cancer (of the bone, I believe), and he was very concerned. I learned later that he never came back to the office after that day, and he died a few weeks later.

Fortunately, situations like the two just mentioned do not occur often, but when they do, our compassion, sympathy, empathy, and most other emotions are called into play. We are constantly reminded that our role as representative is multifaceted, and we may be called upon to provide moral

support for the physician, as well as help for his patients.

Chapter III

The Patient—The Object of a

Representative's Constant Focus

In recent years, after my early retirement from Merck, I have assumed the role of representative again. This time, I am working for a California-based surgical device company, known as New World Medical, Inc. The primary product of New World Medical, Inc. is a unique valved tube shunt device, a surgical implant for the eye, that is used to treat glaucoma. The Ahmed Glaucoma Valve controls the vast majority of the market for such devices, simply because it has greater patient utility than the older devices.

Knowing that I had a lot of experience and training on the subject of glaucoma, while with Merck, New World Medical sought my help in the introduction and promotion of this unique product. Since my retirement from Merck, my wife and I had been successfully operating our own Promotional Products company, so I wasn't looking for a job. This intrigued me, however, and I couldn't resist the prospect of again contributing, in some small way, to the relief of patients pain and suffering. I was fascinated, also, by how the development of the product came about.

You see, Dr. A. Mateen Ahmed, who holds a Ph.D. Degree in the field of Biomedical Engineering, from the prestigious Indian Institute of Technology in New Delhi, India, received Divine inspiration for the development of this unique product. As I understand it, God revealed his command to Dr. Ahmed through a dream. God revealed the nature of this glaucoma device that he was to develop. When he awoke, the mission was clear, and the rest is history. Regardless of religious belief, no one would doubt his story, if they could see, firsthand, how devoted he is to the Worldwide distribution and use of this unique glaucoma valve, that bears his name.

Interacting Directly With Patients

It has been an inspiration to me, on several occasions, to interact directly with patients, who are contemplating this type of surgery. A number of newspaper articles have appeared across the country, stemming largely from interviews with Glaucoma Specialists at the major medical centers, describing the effectiveness and uniqueness of the Ahmed Glaucoma Valve.

Patients who have glaucoma sometimes call me to get more information on the Ahmed Glaucoma Valve. One lady, from a distant city, had learned about our product from a friend, who had the Ahmed Glaucoma Valve implant surgery at UCLA. This patient seemed genuinely thrilled that she might be able to get control of her disease without the emotional side effects that she had experienced with her multi-drug therapy. She even went so far as to say that she would prefer blindness to those drug side effects! I was amazed that a patient would feel that strongly about present therapy. It was very satisfying to me, however, to help reassure her that alternatives did exist. Drug therapy for glaucoma continues to be a mainstay, but some patients simply require more.

Another lady called me for reassurance, and for the names of some Ophthalmologists/Glaucoma Specialists who were doing this type surgery. Again, it made me feel good to know that I had some small part in helping this patient get the care she needed.

Children Tend To Accept Their Fate In Life Better Than Adults

Perhaps the most touching direct encounter with a patient occurred early in my career as a pharmaceutical representative. Merck had a product, an inhalant, that was considered to be useful for the treatment of Cystic Fibrosis. Cystic Fibrosis is a disease of the pancreas, which often affects children, and usually manifests itself as a serious lung disease. The thick mucous produced in the lungs of these patients is often very difficult to expectorate, causing difficult breathing and frequent infections. The disease is frequently fatal before age 20.

Knowing how serious cystic fibrosis is, and how it frequently affects innocent young children, I was excited about what our product could do for those patients. I made my first call on a pediatrician, who had a very large practice. When I gave her a brief introduction of what I wanted to discuss, she immediately said that she would use the product, if it worked on this little girl that she was to see in the hospital in a few minutes. She only required one thing of me. I had to meet her in the Respiratory Therapy section of the hospital, and observe the procedure. I readily agreed, and fifteen minutes later, I was being introduced to this frail bodied eight or ten year old girl, who showed all the signs of the stress that her disease had placed on her. Even with all that stress, she still had a pleasant smile for me. It's an amazing fact that children seem to accept their fate in life, where many adults would buckle.

The therapist began the treatment right away, and it did seem to help almost immediately. Until you have witnessed something like that, you cannot imagine what a thrill it is to have had a small part in relieving a patient's pain and suffering.

To Treat or Not To Treat

Going back to the Ahmed Glaucoma Valve, another ophthalmologist in a small town in Oklahoma, talks about his relationship with his patients. He said he would normally refer patients in need of implant surgery to a Glaucoma Specialist, almost all of whom are located in the larger cities. The problem is, country people will oftentimes refuse to drive to the "big city" for medical treatment. In that case, he said, it's either treat, or let the patient suffer. In other words, if you don't treat them, they won't get treated.

He did his first implant on such a patient. This was an elderly lady, who had advanced glaucoma, and very little vision out of the eye in question, but she had a constant, severe headache, resulting from the severe intraocular pressure in that eye. The response was dramatic! She said she no longer had the headache that had plagued her for years. The family was also delighted with the response.

The Thrill of Having a Part In The Patient's Recovery

Another dramatic story about a patient with Parkinson's Disease comes to mind. A doctor, in a small town, had a patient who suffered from a severe case of Parkinson's Disease. She was residing in a nursing home, had not spoken a word, or changed her expression for years. When L-DOPA became available, this physician started a course of therapy on this patient. Again, the response was dramatic! She began speaking again, and was soon able to go home. Great news for the treating physician and the patient, but all was not well, when the patient got home. You see, family members, who thought, if Grandma couldn't speak, she also could not hear. It seems that several family members had made comments about her, while she was in the nursing home, that they wished now they hadn't. They eventually ironed out that rough spot, but something more serious happened. It seems that L-DOPA, as wonderful as it was at first, started to lose it's effectiveness. It had something to do with the ability to get dopamine, the active ingredient of L-DOPA, across the blood brain barrier, without first being destroyed.

About that time, Merck released a product known generically as Carbidopa-Levodopa. This product promised to solve the blood brain barrier problem of L-DOPA, and it's use still continues. The patient just described, had a renewed response on Carbidopa-Levodopa, and went on to live a normal life. Again, it was quite a thrill to me to have had some small part in this patient's favorable outcome, through my introduction of Merck's new product to that physician.

The Patient Instructor

At one time in my career as a representative, I was involved in the introduction and promotion of a small group of products specifically indicated for the treatment of arthritis and other musculoskeletal disorders. During this time, I was introduced to one of the most unique patient oriented programs I have ever seen. The program originated at the University of Arizona, under the direction of one of the rheumatologists on the faculty there. This rheumatologist discovered that patients with severe rheumatoid arthritis were willing to volunteer their time, and considerable effort, to help train other newly diagnosed RA patients how best to manage their disease. Another interesting discovery was that these volunteers saw a decrease in symptoms from their own disease, because of their involvement in this program.

I was privileged to be a part of a training class where these patient volunteers were brought in to help representatives gain a better understanding of rheumatoid arthritis from the patient's perspective. This was a hands-on session, and really drove home the age old Merck philosophy expressed by George W. Merck in the following statement:

"We try never to forget that medicine is for the people. It is not for the profits. The profits follow, and if we have remembered that, they have never failed to appear."

I don't know if this program is still in existence or not. I sincerely hope so, and if not, I would hope it would be reactivated. Sponsorship of a program of this type would also be a very worthwhile endeavor for a pharmaceutical or medical device company.

Mentors

Over the past several years, I have developed a close working relationship with another very important person in my understanding of the challenges the Glaucoma Specialist faces, and how these challenges affect the patient. The person I am referring to is William E. Sponsel, M.D., Director of Clinical Research, Department of Ophthalmology, Glaucoma Section, The University of Texas Health Science Center at San Antonio. He and I have spent many hours discussing this subject. These discussions have been especially helpful to me, because Doctor Sponsel has a greater depth of understanding than most about why, as well as what, things occur during the course of treatment for glaucoma. His research, coupled with his surgery, makes the patient response more predictable. Doctor Sponsel also has a greater depth of understanding about the complications that sometimes occur with tube shunts in general. For instance, he not only knows that complications occur occasionally, but his research suggests ways of managing post-surgical complications, so that the patient is not denied the benefits of the device.

I feel privileged to have had a roll in helping Doctor Sponsel plan several seminars for ophthalmologists across the Country, who seek a better understanding of the treatment of glaucoma. These seminars have been well attended, and again, the patient is the beneficiary.

The knowledge I gain from my discussions with Doctor Sponsel is very valuable to me, as I carry on discussions with other ophthalmologists. Everyone needs a mentor, and I consider Doctor Sponsel my mentor. You too, should seek out someone in your own area that you have good rapport with, and one that is willing to serve as your mentor.

Just as Art Linkletter saw in children;

"Patients Say The Darndest Things"

The following is a true story, as told by one of my competitors. My competitor was waiting, in the waiting room, to see the doctors in this small town clinic. The clinic had picked that day to carry out their annual flu immunization program. My competitor witnesses the following scenario: This patient walks in, goes up to the reception office, and declares that he wants to get a "flu shot". The receptionist told him to have a seat, and the nurse would call him in a minute. As the patient sits down

31

near my competitor, he says; "This is the worst case of flu I've had in years! Through this misunderstanding, the patient is about to receive a shot to <u>prevent</u> flu, when what he wants is a shot to <u>treat</u> flu. What would you do, if you witnessed something like this? Here's what my competitor felt obligated to do, for the benefit of the patient. He quietly, and politely, went back into the clinic hallway, and discretely revealed to the nurse what he had witnessed. Needless to say, the nurse was grateful for the information, and my competitor felt that he had done his duty to the patient.

Chapter IV

Co-Workers—Teamwork is Essential

For many years, pharmaceutical/medical representatives worked pretty much in isolation. They worked large territories, and rarely saw their peers, except at meetings. That has all changed now. Most pharmaceutical companies have multiple sales forces, and as many as twenty, thirty, or more representatives, where one or two used to be the norm. With more and more representatives promoting more and more groups of products, teamwork is an absolute essential, if the Company and the representative are to optimize the return on their efforts and investment.

Teamwork Made The Difference

Several years back, Merck was faced with a large number of important products, and the realization that one representative in each area could no longer do an adequate job of promoting that many products at one time. Other companies faced a similar dilemma, but Merck was the first to act on it. Split the product line, and create a second sales force, seemed to be the appropriate solution. I was pleased to be a part of one of the first test areas.

Since this approach had never been tried in the pharmaceutical industry, no one knew what the reaction might be, between the different members of the sales force. As a result, promotion of teamwork was a top priority.

The following year, it was my privilege, again, to be selected to present my findings and recommendations on the subject to a neighboring Region. The following, slightly abridged, text of that speech best expresses my views:

The Responsibility For Teamwork Belongs To All Members of The Sales Team

As a member of a neighboring Region, I have had the opportunity of participating for the past year in the testing of a unique, innovative, and highly successful new program, which is embodied in the two groups that you are already familiar with.

I've been asked to come here today, and share some of my thoughts and experiences with you, so that you might have a better understanding of what you are about to become a part of.

Regardless of your position in this Region, you will soon be entering one of the most exciting eras of your career. I say this without reservation, and without regard to any particular job or group within your Region. Regardless of the group you are in, you are as much a part of this exciting new era as anyone else in your Region.

It is my firm conviction that the responsibility, and indeed the credit, for the success of this new program rests equally on each and every member of the Region.

This new organization makes situations commonplace, that never before existed in the majority of territories. Some of you will likely be working in close harmony with as many as three, or perhaps four other representatives. A large part of the excitement is getting to know these other representatives, and sharing with them your day-to-day and week-to-week experiences.

You may say to yourself that you already know the other representatives you'll be working with, but believe me, you can't really appreciate another representative until you've had the pleasure of working in close harmony with them. I can speak from experience—I was in the same District three years with the three representatives in my area, prior to joining the new group. I was certain I knew them pretty well, and as we all do, had a number of preconceived ideas about how they might react to my presence in "their territory". To make a long story short, I realized immediately that I really didn't know them as well as I thought I did. To my very pleasant surprise, they welcomed me with open arms.

What I'm saying is simply this—Don't waste any time in getting to know your fellow representatives. I urge each and every one of you to take the initiative in welcoming, and getting acquainted with each of the representatives in your area. Get together for several hours prior to making any calls. Find out as much as you can about each other, as you go over the geography and physician population of your new area. If you are the host, take your counterpart for a get-acquainted drive around town—have lunch at your favorite spot. These things may seem trivial, but they all tend to make you feel more like a team.

If there are any key words to describe what is necessary to maximize your enjoyment of your job, and help the program achieve it's highest potential, they would be sincerity, diplomacy, finesse, common courtesy, and above all, cooperation.

One of the things that we've found to be very helpful to us is to communicate freely and frequently. Call your teammates up, or drop them a note, often. Just as a rule of thumb, don't let a week go by, without some contact. We sometimes confer with each other two or three times a week, frequently, but not always, about business matters. The main thing is to maintain almost constant contact.

Many are the ways that you can help your counterpart, and they in turn, can do the same for you. Exchanging information on competitive activities in our territories is a classic example.

We quite often take care of a physician's or clinic's sample needs for each other. If a physician asks me for samples of another group's, for instance, I simply tell him/her that that is one of Al's, Bob's, or Paul's products, but I will ask them to see that he gets what he needs, if he will just sign the appropriate card. When I leave his office, I fill out the appropriate documents, and go ahead and send the physician whatever is needed. The other representatives do the same for me. This way, the physician gets what he wants without delay, and the image of all our representatives is enhanced. It has been helpful to know when this has happened, and this is the type information that we exchange frequently.

If at all possible, a visit with your counterpart over breakfast or lunch two or three times a month is a great idea. We use this time to exchange information relating to new accounts, changes in account buying status, new physicians in the area, physicians leaving the area, physicians who have died, specific physician comments about our activities, and various other bits of information that we think would be helpful.

I feel that one word of caution is in order—Be helpful in every way that you can, but avoid at all costs any chance of interference in the operation of another representative's territory. If you will do that, the lines of communication will stay open, and the spirit of cooperation will prevail.

It has been very helpful to us to do long-range planning of physician conferences together. We make every effort to attend each other's conferences, and look forward to sharing the other representative's company and support at these meetings. This seems to cause the physician to think of us as a team, and a visit in their office by either of us tends to reinforce the efforts of the other. Again, common courtesy is the rule, when we attend another representative's conference. We try to avoid interfering with the meeting in any way. In other words, we try to conduct ourselves as the guest that we are.

Hospital and clinic displays are yet another area where joint effort seems to be very effective. Side by side, my counterparts and I sometimes conduct hospital displays, and also clinic displays for our residents. This is not a chance meeting. We have a prearranged plan to do just that. In this setting, we play host for each other—introducing our counterpart to those physicians that maybe we have met, and the other representative hasn't. In this way, any good will that is created by either representative, with a physician that has been difficult for the other representative to see, is shared by both representatives.

In a similar fashion, my friends from the other groups and I have worked exhibits at small medical meetings— each representative working his own group of products right out of the same booth.

You may think you're pretty effective alone in your territory—I did—and I know for a fact that you are, but don't underestimate the power of teamwork!

I'm convinced that we have accomplished things working together that might never have been accomplished by any representative working alone. One physician in my territory was widely known to be an absolute refusal for all pharmaceutical company representatives, and continues to be for other companies. He responded cautiously, but positively, to our approach as a team, and has been receptive to both representatives ever since.

The representative in the same area introduced me to his "back door" privilege for the local rheumatologist, a very busy and influential physician, who practices in a relatively "closed" clinic, as far as conventional detailing is concerned. This bit of assistance has saved me months, or perhaps years, of time and effort. As a result, I have had easy access to this important physician, with very little time invested. Again, teamwork made the difference.

Directors of Medical Education have also been very responsive to the team approach. They have been very willing to let each of us schedule programs on an alternate basis, where they had shown resistance to even one program in the past. They seem to pay more attention to what we have to offer, when approached by two representatives, instead of one.

To summarize briefly, it would benefit you, your associates, and the Company, if, as soon as you know who the representatives are, that you will be working with, you would:

1. Waste no time in contacting those representatives, offering your help, and soliciting theirs.

2. Arrange for a meeting of a half a day or so with the representatives involved, to exchange territorial information, and to get to know each other.

3. Share your "trade secrets" with your counterparts—Help them to enjoy the same privileges you do.

4. Be supportive of your fellow associates. Shower them with all the information and help you can muster—You will each be better off for it.

5. Keep in touch—Communicate at least once a week.

6. Remember always the terms sincerity, diplomacy, finesse, common courtesy, and above all, cooperation.

Thank you for letting me share these thoughts with you—Good luck, and smooth sailing!

Co-Workers As Mentors

Just as Doctor Sponsel serves as my unofficial mentor now, every small group of representatives, whether it be called District, Region, or whatever, has one or two co-workers, who serve as excellent mentors. For the first several years of my career, I was blessed to have in my District, a man who stood head and shoulders above most other representatives—a man of great stature and values, that most of us only dream of. This person was assigned to a large military territory with management level status. He operated more or less autonomously, but was assigned to my District for administrative purposes only. He always attended our District meetings, and what a contribution he did make! I learned so much from this individual. I consider him, to this day, one of my greatest mentors. My life has been enriched by the influence of this great man.

Look for someone like this to help guide you in your career.

Chapter V

Competitors—Friend or Foe?

Some companies frown on their representatives getting friendly with their competitors. I think this is something that has to be at the discretion of the representative. After all, a competitor introduced me to my wife, and I will be forever grateful for that. My wife and this competitor's wife were longtime friends and roommates, after they graduated from college. This competitor and I became the best of friends, but we were fierce competitors on the territory. There are areas of most territories that require rather lengthy waits, and oftentimes you find yourself in the company of one, or several competitors. You get to know these people pretty well, and you soon learn who to be friendly with, and who to not be friendly with.

The company's concern, always, is that you might be drawn into a discussion of prices, etc., which of course is illegal, and can cause a company a lot of grief. I always keep my distance from such discussions, but there are often other things that might be discussed that are very helpful. For instance, doctors who have moved recently, or personnel changes at hospitals or pharmacies, that might be helpful to know in advance.

I had very good rapport with my competitors in my first territory. This turned out to be real helpful at one point. I don't know if you have ever had the mumps, but I did, when our children were about two and three. I was flat of my back in bed for three weeks, because of the usual complications. After the first week and a half, my wife joined me, also with a complicated case of the mumps.

So, what does this have to do with my competitors, you say? The day before I was diagnosed, I was visiting with a couple of competitors on the parking lot of this large clinic. I rubbed my jaw and neck, and jokingly commented that I thought I was getting the mumps. Both my competitors disappeared under a nearby car, where I heard loud voices say, "Oh, my God! I haven't had the mumps either!" I tried to reassure them, but to no avail, so I got in my car and went on home. It was no joke the next day, I assure you.

Good Rapport Pays Off

Getting back to my competitors, and how my rapport with them paid off. Word got around almost immediately (probably through my doctor) that I was in bed with the mumps. After a few days, many of my competitors started collecting questions and requests from my doctors, and even passed on orders from hospitals and pharmacies to me. I was overwhelmed and humbled by the experience. I never would have expected such generous support. It made going back to work so much easier.

Another example of a friendly competitor that made many long days easier, was a representative of another major company. He and I seemed to arrive regularly at this large clinic, in not-so-large a town, on the same day. After waiting in the hallway all morning, as we usually did, we often had a leisurely lunch at the Thunderbird Motel Restaurant. We usually ordered the Chef's Salad, so we could pretend we had eaten, and still not gain any weight. Invariably, this representative and I would get into a discussion involving our churches, and religion in general. It was, we thought a highly intellectual discussion, and reminded both of us of our lives in the college dorm.

We seldom solved the problem of the day, but we went back to work after lunch much more relaxed than when we arrived there. I'm sure our productivity was enhanced by this brief respite.

The summation is, you pick competitors to be friendly with, just like you would pick any other friend. Mutual respect and trust are the keys.

Chapter VI

Pharmacists and Their Changing Role

Retail pharmacists are playing an ever declining role in the management of a representative's territory. Except for very small towns, independent pharmacies are almost a thing of the past. Large chains, such as Walgreen's or Rite Aid, are the rule, rather than the exception. Many pharmacists have become somewhat hostile toward pharmaceutical companies and their representatives, because of what they consider as infringements on their turf.

Managed Health Care and Hospital Pharmacists Play A Larger Role

HMO and hospital pharmacists are an entirely different matter. This group of pharmacists still has tremendous influence on which drugs their patients will have access to. Regular contact with this group has become more and more important, because they exert tremendous influence on what drugs will be permitted on their formulary.

Various forms of statistical data on the prescribing habits of physicians is now available to pharmaceutical companies, so informal collection of that information from the corner pharmacy is less important.

With surgical devices, most of the influence in any given hospital, or surgery center, is through the surgeon and the OR supervisors. Key considerations here are whether insurance or Medicare/Medicaid will pay for it. Most

hospitals require clearance through Purchasing, before a

representative is allowed to visit Surgery or the OR

(Operating Room).

Chapter VII

Nurses/Assistants

Never to be overlooked, or taken lightly, are the physician's nurses or assistants (office assistant, surgical assistant, secretary, technician, etc.). I have found that it is very helpful for me to get to know as many people as I can, that work in close harmony with the physician. This group of associates share much of the physician's concern for the patient, and they are acutely aware of the most appropriate time for the representative to visit. If the office staff readily recognizes you, when you call for an appointment, they tend to knock themselves out to help you. I frequently call ahead to let them know I will be there on a certain day, even if I don't have a specific appointment. I've found that it really helps, if I am able to tell the secretary, "Doctor _____" is expecting me.

It Is Helpful To Know What Pleases or Displeases The Physician

Members of the physician's staff sometimes confide in the representative some of the things that please, or displease, their doctor, when a representative calls on them. This is very valuable information, in view of the fact that one always hopes to please. Developing good rapport with the physician's staff is a win, win situation.

Chapter VIII

Managers and Their Representatives

The Manager, Who Manages Least, Manages Best

It has been said that the manager who manages least, manages best. An astute manager realizes that leadership is what it's all about. A pharmaceutical/medical manager must LEAD, not DRIVE the representative. The concept of chain of command must be understood, and abided by. The representative's success, and indeed, livelihood, depends on the manager's ability to interpret the representative to the manager's superiors.

Historic Perspective

The representative must realize that they have the responsibility of interpreting themselves, and their accomplishments, to their manager. When a representative is assigned to a new manager, it behooves that representative to present the new manager with a historic perspective on his/her career. This should read somewhat like a lengthy resume. It should contain all the major assignments, and achievements, in your career to date. It is useful, also, to include one's goals and ambitions for the future. You would be amazed at how many representatives are approaching retirement, before their manager finds out that they have been interested for years in getting into management. Somehow or other, they must think their manager gets such information by OSMOSIS! This document is perhaps the most important of one's career. The Historic Perspective provides a clear understanding of where the representative has been, as well as where the representative wants to go. The representative should have the Historic Perspective prepared, and ready to present, at their first one-on-one meeting with their new manager. Careful attention to neatness and form are essential.

Management Position Is Not For Everyone

Some representatives get the impression that they are expected to aspire to a position in management, if they are to succeed in their career. Success doesn't necessarily include promotion to manager. If one is prepared for management, and really wants to be a manager of people, then they should go for it. On the other hand, if one does not have special management skills, or real interest in managing people, they should consider going the route of field promotion, and remain on the territory. Most companies nowadays have a range of promotions available to representatives, where they get special recognition and increased pay, but remain on the territory. A full, complete, productive, and satisfying career on the territory is entirely possible. The special talents of many of these representatives should be utilized by their manager. This re-emphasizes their value as a representative, and also keeps interest up. Participation in special projects would be a classic example.

Pistol on The Hip Syndrome

Every company has, at some time or other, promoted some individuals to management, that should not have been managers. Because these individuals are not equipped to handle the responsibility that has been bestowed upon them, they develop an inflated opinion of their importance. I liken this to the "good ol' boy" in a small western town, that one day became a deputy sheriff. The pistol on the hip immediately went to his head, and he spent the rest of his days making those around him miserable—thus, "pistol on the hip syndrome".

There is somehow the misguided perception by some inexperienced managers, that to maintain control, one must not allow themselves to be friendly, or too well liked, by the people they supervise. They let their ego cloud their good judgement. Mutual respect and admiration between manager and representative is a far more formidable force, than an atmosphere of fear and distrust.

As almost everyone will agree, the best managers are mild mannered, very intelligent, very tolerant, and basically very nice people to be around. Their most notable feature is that they are constantly ASKING, rather than TELLING. The astute manager is a staunch advocate for his/her representatives. To solve problems, they create an atmosphere whereby the representative will usually be able to solve their own problems. They ask lots of questions, and offer a number of possible solutions. In this manner, the representative's feeling of self reliance is enhanced. If, and only if, all else fails, the astute manager is then prepared to "take the bull by the horns".

The Work Performance Review, Performance Appraisal, Performance Review, or Whatever Your Company Calls It

The annual performance appraisal is perhaps the most important document of your career. The resume' may get you the job, but the annual appraisal determines everything about your career, from that moment on—salary increases, bonuses, stock options, participation in special projects, promotions, and much more. Managers don't "GIVE" you anything, you have to "EARN IT THE OLD FASHIONED WAY" —hard work!

The annual review is not intended to be one sided. The sooner one learns that this is a participative session, the better off they will be.

Write Your Own Review/Appraisal

Very early on, I realized that my manager was not always aware of something I did, that would have a marked impact on the rating I would get on my appraisal. I started then to prepare my own performance review, with the supporting documents for each category of the review. This always "blew the mind" of my manager, when we sat down for the first appraisal together. I didn't quite understand this, because I always thought it was my responsibility to appraise my performance myself, in order to be prepared to participate in the appraisal by my manager. I am convinced that I got better appraisals through the years because of this, and I would strongly recommend that you do the same.

My last District Manager, before I retired from Merck, was perhaps the best at doing Work Performance Reviews.

She was very thorough in her preparation, and was always willing to concede a point, if I had documented evidence that I deserved a better rating. I've talked to many other representatives through the years, and most went to the appraisal session totally unprepared to participate. They oftentimes spent the whole day arguing uselessly that they deserved a better rating. You see, they had no DOCUMENTED evidence, to back up their claim.

What lawyer, worth his salt, would go to court without preparing his case? I think it is basically a fair comparison—PREPARE NOT, WIN NOT!

Getting back to my last District Manager with Merck. She knew I was prepared to support my position, so she went through each point, presented her rating in each category, and I in turn, presented mine. If I had documented evidence that she had failed to note, or was unaware of, she changed the rating accordingly. I considered this to be very fair and equitable, and it always buoyed my enthusiasm for the next year.

Helpful Hints For Better Ratings

Following are some helpful hints on how to consistently get higher ratings on the Performance Appraisal:

1) The annual performance appraisal is ongoing. Start preparation for next year's appraisal as soon as this year's appraisal is completed. Don't wait until the last minute—That's too late!

2) Think of the appraisal as a building block process for career development.

3) Strive for consistent ratings, preferably with an upward trend. This is very important, when being considered for a raise or promotion.

4) Plan activities early in the appraisal period that will enhance performance, and ratings will reflect your effort. Keep your manager informed of what you're doing, and KEEP GOOD RECORDS.

5) Go to the appraisal session well prepared. Here's where the good records you have kept all year will really pay off. Organize your records of accomplishments to coincide with the element of the review or appraisal that it relates to. For example, the achievement of an objective should coincide with the element "Achievement of Objectives".

6) Consider writing your own Appraisal/Review using the format of the form that is customarily used by

your company. Write the appraisal, as you see it, and include all the supporting data for each element.

NOTE TO MANAGERS: If a representative's performance on a given element EXCEEDS EXPECTIONS, it should be so noted. Some managers use the excuse that they don't give anyone a higher rating than MEETS EXPECTIONS, but that is little comfort to the representative, who has clearly exceeded expectations. This does not necessarily mean that the overall rating will be different, but simply means that credit should be given, where credit is due.

7) Be as objective as possible. Be specific about accomplishments, using exact numbers and dates, if

possible. This will be possible, only if you keep good records.

8) In setting your goals for the next appraisal period, be specific in outlining your goals. Make sure they are attainable, measurable, and contain some stretch (challenge).

9) Work WITH, not AGAINST, your manager. Don't hesitate to ask what is required of you to reach a desired goal.

10) Ask your manager to help you formulate a long-range plan, and the specific goals necessary to achieve the desired level. Perhaps you want to work toward a field promotion to Senior Representative, or maybe you want to get into field management, or the Training Department. Whatever your interests are, be as specific as possible.

11) Keep in mind always that PROMOTIONS ARE BASED ON SUPERIOR PERFORMANCE IN YOUR PRESENT POSITION. You are not likely to be promoted to a higher level, unless you are doing an outstanding job at your current level. That's just the way the system works. PROMOTIONS ARE DESIGNED TO REWARD ACHIEVEMENT.

As you have probably gathered by now, I've had experience working for more than the usual number of managers during the course of my career, so there is not much that I have not witnessed. I am particularly indebted to two particular District Managers, who helped lead me in the right direction to achieve important goals. One of these managers followed one of those managers that I described earlier. The new manager was just out of a management position in Sales Training, and was like a breath of fresh air for me. We always had a great time, when he traveled with me. We were constantly bouncing ideas off each other, and he was very effective in encouraging me to read books on communications skills. Unfortunately, I was transferred out of his District after a year or so, but he continued to be a strong influence on my career.

The other District Manager came to my District while I was working on my field promotion to the Executive level. He taught me a great deal about setting goals and achieving objectives. He saw me through this promotion, and I will always be grateful to him for that. Without his generous input on setting goals and achieving objectives, I might never have succeeded in reaching that highest level of achievement. He was later promoted to a Home Office position, and will always be a true friend and advocate.

Guidelines For The RepresentativeIn His/Her Relationship With Their Manager

The following are some areas of great importance in the relationship of the representative with their manager:

1) Timely Reporting

   Reports required by the Company, or the manager, should always be submitted in a timely manner. You might say that this goes without saying, but you would be surprised how many representatives fail to do this, creating the manager's worst nightmare.

   One of the primary responsibilities of a representative is to keep management informed.

This should be ongoing, and greatly enhances your image with your manager.

2) Keep Communications Channels Open

Representatives, as well as managers, should always strive to keep communications flowing. Neither functions with great efficiency in the dark. The mutual benefit here is obvious.

3) Neatness

This may sound like a third grade point, but is soooo important. Paperwork should be typed, autos should be kept clean and well maintained, and presentations at meetings should show signs of preparation.

4) Willingness To Share

Willingness to share skills and information with peers is an important function for the successful representative. Managers should encourage, and expect, this of their representatives.

5) Flexibility

Willingness to be flexible is another characteristic that will help the representative get high marks. Changing one's schedule, to accommodate a request of the manager, is a good example.

6) Achievement of Sales Objectives

The representative should always be aware of, and supportive of management's goals. If special support is needed to achieve sales objectives, the representative should make such requests early. Managers seldom penalize a representative for not achieving sales objectives, if the representative has utilized all the sales support available to them. This is one place, where good records documenting every detail, is essential.

My Theory of The Declining Circle

A phenomena that I discovered early on in my career is what I refer to as "The Theory of The Declining Circle". I have described this theory to many new representatives, who later thanked me for saving them from falling into that trap. So, what is the theory? When a new representative goes on territory, they have a tendency to leave no stone unturned. They call on virtually everyone, to carryout their mission for the patient. They make a big circle of their territory. As they grow "smarter", they decide that some of those they have been calling on represent a smaller contribution to their sales effort. Selective promotion sets in, and they reduce the size of their "circle". This continues until the circle of prospects is at it's "optimal" size—thus the "Theory of The Declining Circle".

The irony is, most new representatives show their most dramatic growth in sales during that first few months to a year, when their circle of coverage is largest. As the circle declines, so does the sales growth. Complete coverage of the territory, I've discovered, is always the most productive, provided you don't neglect the doctors with the highest potential, who are sometimes harder to see. I understand the concept of TARGETING, but I believe one can do both.

"See The People"

To emphasize the point that you have to make the calls, one learned representative in my first District, told the story of the clown, who looked out over the vast audience and said, "See the people, see the people". That's what you have to do to excel—See the people!

7) Don't Burn Bridges

Sometimes, when a representative undergoes a change of manager, a change of the company they work for, or some other momentous event in their career, they are inclined to want to get a lot of things off their chest. Don't give in to that temptation! That will only be perceived as "sour grapes", and will not enhance your image or career. Always present the appearance of running TO something, instead of running FROM something. In other words, be positive about the future, and let the past take care of itself.

8) Career Goals

The representative should have well planned and clearly stated goals. The manager must understand clearly what you want from your career. You may want more than the manager can get for you, but a clear understanding is essential.

A Word About The Manager's Demeanor

It was always apparent to me, that a manager who was fun to work with seemed to accomplish more. A little levity now and then helps lighten the load. From the archives of my mind, I recall one particular instance that rekindled a smile for years thereafter. Following the release meeting for an important new product, my District Manager informed his District members that they should "keep an eye out for him", because he was planning a whirlwind visit with each member, during the following two weeks. When he arrived for his brief visit with me, we got in my car, and I handed him an eye model (a carryover from a previous promotion). What's this, he asked? When I reminded him that he ask us to keep an eye out for him, he burst into laughter, and we shared the laughter with others for years thereafter.

Perhaps this is a trivial example, but characterized the fun we had when we worked together, and it made us look forward to, rather than dread, those times.

I've heard it said that success does not always breed happiness. In my experience, a happy work environment does breed success.

Chapter IX

Summary

The following describes what I would consider the representatives never ending goal:

You have to shoot for the moon—If you miss, you'll still be among the stars!

Success and happiness are not necessarily the same, but careful attention to the suggestions and observations offered in this book, will enhance the probability that you, the representative, will enjoy more of both.

We have discussed the philosophy of focusing on the patient's needs, the role of the physician and the development of a mutual trust and respect, the all important patient as the constant focus, co-workers as mentors, and the need for teamwork, competitors and the contribution they can make, pharmacists and their changing role, nurses and assistants and the important role they play, and the extensive role that managers play in our quest for success and happiness.

As one who is pursuing his third career, I have learned a lot from my experience, and I sincerely hope that sharing my experiences and observations, as a representative, will help you to become a more effective representative, in a shorter period of time.

I urge you to never lose sight of the primary focus—that all important patient.

Good luck and Best wishes.

About the Author

Travis E. Doss graduated Cum Laude from Baylor University, with a BBA Degree in Management. He attended The University of Texas College of Pharmacy, and did graduate work in Marketing at Baylor University.

Mr. Doss is a life member of Beta Gamma Sigma, and Alpha Chi. He has been the recipient of numerous District, Region, and National Sales Awards.

Mr. Doss began his career in 1959, as a Professional Representative with Merck. He was promoted in 1978 to Senior Professional Representative, with Merck's Human Health Division, and to Executive Professional Representative in 1983.

Mr. Doss was certified by Merck in 1983, as a Qualified Counselor for purposes of counseling and training. He has served as counselor or trainer for numerous training classes. He was selected by his Region Manager to participate in several pilot projects, such as Merck's Clinical Conference Program, and the first rollout of a new sales force.

In 1989, Mr. Doss was selected by his Region Manager to serve on the Region Manager's Advisory Committee. In 1990, Mr. Doss took early retirement from Merck, and he and his wife were co-owners of Dunraven's Advertising Specialties, until 1997.

Since 1995, Mr. Doss has served as Sales Representative for New World Medical, Inc., who develops, manufactures, and markets surgical devices, used in the treatment of Glaucoma.

www.ingramcontent.com/pod-product-compliance
Lightning Source LLC
Chambersburg PA
CBHW030105300526
45785CB00019B/1793